"What a pleasure to read! This book has 100 sleep tips, presented in a clear, consistent, easy-to-read and completely non-judgemental way. These qualities make it the children's sleep guide you can trust – dipping into it anytime and coming away with realistic advice that you can start to put into practice right there and then. It is written by an author who is absolutely dedicated in her support for parents, who has years of experience both professionally and personally and who reassuringly understands how the science of sleep impacts and influences every one of the sleep tips she shares."

Dr Ella Rachamim, paediatrician, author and director of Be Ready to Parent (www.bereadytoparent.com)

"This is such a great resource for new parents to help them and their babies get the best sleep possible. A really well laid out series of sensible and easy to implement tips from an expert in her field. It will help parents navigate through the early days getting good sleep habits right from day one and then to help avoid the common pitfalls as the baby gets older. A must-have read for new parents."

Beth Graham, midwife and lactation consultant www.midwifebeth.com

100 TIPS TO HELP YOUR BABY SLEEP

An Hachette UK Company
www.hachette.co.uk

Vie Books, an imprint of Summersdale Publishers Ltd
Part of Octopus Publishing Group Limited
Carmelite House
50 Victoria Embankment
LONDON
EC4Y 0DZ
UK

www.summersdale.com

Printed and bound in China

ISBN: 978-1-78685-984-6

Substantial discounts on bulk quantities of Summersdale books are available to corporations, professional associations and other organizations. For details contact general enquiries: telephone: +44 (0) 1243 771107 or email: enquiries@summersdale.com.

Disclaimer: The information given in this book should not be treated as a substitute for qualified medical advice. Neither the author nor the publisher can be held responsible for any loss or claim arising out of the use, or misuse, of the suggestions made or the failure to take medical advice.

100
TIPS

TO HELP YOUR
BABY SLEEP

STEPHANIE MODELL

AUTHOR OF THE BESTSELLING *THE BABY SLEEP GUIDE*

CONTENTS

INTRODUCTION

Since writing my first book, *The Baby Sleep Guide*, in 2015, I have received so many kind emails and reviews saying how it has helped families to enjoy their babies due to a good night's sleep. It's a straightforward, honest book that makes no false promises. My aim was to deliver sleep education so parents would have knowledge about how babies sleep and their patterns and rhythms without having to trawl through hundreds of pages of complicated information.

However, in an ever-increasingly technical world where we are bombarded with information yet are time poor, *100 Tips to Help Your Baby Sleep* offers the most succinct advice in bite-size tips that can be read in an instant and acted upon easily.

By following the simple tips within this book, you will learn how your baby's sleep patterns can be slowly and gently moulded to suit your family's lifestyle. By providing consistent positive cues at bedtime and naptime along with reassurance, your baby will learn to associate these cues with sleep and will learn to fall asleep unassisted, the benefits of which will be a good night's sleep for all, and a happy, contented baby.

Enjoy!

NOTES FROM THE AUTHOR

- Even though this is a book about sleep, I'm also going to focus on feeding. A hungry baby will be unsettled and is unlikely to sleep!

- Every baby is different, as are parenting styles, but I am confident that you will find helpful ways to establish positive sleep habits for your baby within these pages.

- I would also like to add that this is not about "training" your baby to sleep. Sleep is an automatic behaviour triggered by the build-up of sleep pressure. Foetuses sleep *in utero* with no learning involved. However, falling asleep in response to external (the carer's) cues rather than internal biological cues is a learned behaviour.

- If your baby is sleeping during the day and is wide awake at night, parents may understandably feel that they are doing something wrong or that there is something wrong with their baby, but if you anticipate the fact that your baby's inherent biology may not be in tune with modern lifestyles you will find ways of coping with this initial imbalance.

- It is fair to say that some babies are easier than others. Some are described as "fussy" babies or colicky babies, while some are relaxed and easy-going from the outset and as long as they are well fed they sleep. In this book I am not able to cover medical issues but if your baby gets particularly distressed in a way that is beyond fussiness, you need to seek professional help to rule out a medical problem, such as a milk allergy or intolerance, reflux or silent reflux, which can be particularly hard to diagnose.

- Statistics on global sleep deprivation and its impact on our mental and physical health and productivity are well documented, and some forward-thinking doctors have even begun prescribing sleep to patients in place of medicine. By establishing positive sleep habits early on, you will be providing your baby with the best start and instilling a vital life skill.

- This book is not in chronological order and some of the tips will differ according to the age of your baby. I have tried to accommodate this where necessary; however, I would suggest that you initially read the tips from start to finish and then refer back as required.

- I have chosen to refer to your baby as "she" throughout the book to avoid sounding impersonal. However, clearly, my advice is for all babies, male and female.

SAFE SLEEP

B abies need a lot of sleep during the first few months of their lives so it's important to ensure that they are sleeping as safely as possible. Sudden infant death syndrome (SIDS) is the sudden and unexplained death of a baby where no cause is found. While SIDS is rare, it can still happen and there are steps that parents can take to help reduce the chance of this tragedy occurring. The Lullaby Trust is a British charitable organization that's considered the recognized national authority on safe sleeping practices for infants and children. They recommend that parents follow their advice (below) to significantly reduce the risk of SIDS. Aim to follow the advice for all sleep periods, not just at night.

Things you can do:

- Always place your baby on their back to sleep, with their feet positioned at the bottom of the cot.

- Keep your baby smoke-free during pregnancy and after birth.

- Place your baby to sleep in a separate cot or Moses basket in the same room as you for the first 6 months.

- Breastfeed your baby if you can.

- Use a firm, flat, waterproof mattress that's in good condition.

  Things to avoid:

- Never sleep on a sofa or in an armchair with your baby as this increases the risk of SIDS dramatically.
- Don't sleep in the same bed as your baby if you smoke, drink or take drugs, are extremely tired, or if your baby was born prematurely or was of low birth weight.
- Avoid letting your baby get too hot.
- Don't cover your baby's face or head while sleeping or use loose bedding or pillows.

More information can be found at www.lullabytrust.org.uk.

I feel it's important to say here that some parents choose to co-sleep. If this is your choice, please seek advice from your midwife, health visitor or paediatrician on how to do this in the safest way possible. The most dangerous time to co-sleep is if it's done through exhaustion rather than choice.

CHAPTER 1

UNDERSTANDING SLEEP

INTRODUCTION

Understanding *how* babies sleep is essential to help encourage a good night's sleep. This section explains the biology of sleep, sleep cycles, sleep hormones and your baby's sleep patterns over 24 hours. Once you have this overall picture you will be able to establish positive sleep habits from the outset, which will help to avoid the necessity of sleep training further down the line.

1.

UNDERSTAND THE BENEFITS OF POSITIVE SLEEP HABITS

Sleep is essential for the physical and psychological health of your baby or child. Studies have proven that a good night's sleep and regular bedtime routine have a significantly positive impact on a child's:

- Well-being
- Health
- Behaviour
- Memory
- Ability to learn.

Lack of sleep has been linked with obesity, aggression, behavioural problems, low IQ and poor memory. Sleep deprivation has a negative impact on the whole family and sleep-deprived parents can find positive parenting challenging.

2.

AVERAGE SLEEP NEEDS CHART

This chart shows the "average" sleep needs of a baby or child; however, please bear in mind that "average" can vary greatly between babies, so only refer to this as a guide.

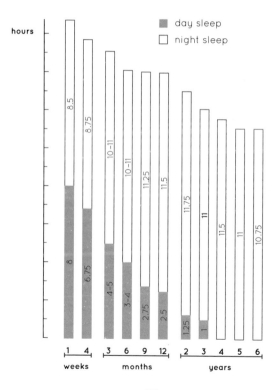

17

3.

LEARN ABOUT THE DIFFERENT TYPES OF SLEEP

When we go to sleep it's not a simple matter of switching off and then waking up in the morning: we go through cycles, experiencing various stages along the way, from drowsiness to light sleep, to slow-wave deep sleep and dream sleep. Even though your body is resting and restoring its energy levels, sleep is an active state that's essential for your physical and mental well-being.

We can divide sleep into two broad types: non-rapid eye movement (NREM) sleep and rapid eye movement (REM) sleep. In order to feel well rested and be in good health both physically and mentally, we need to achieve an adequate amount of both types of sleep during the night.

4.

NREM SLEEP (NON-RAPID EYE MOVEMENT SLEEP)

Deep NREM sleep, also known as stage 3 sleep, is when the brain rests, blood is released to the muscles, energy is restored, tissue is grown or repaired, hormones are released for growth and development, and the immune system is strengthened. During NREM sleep your baby will breathe steadily and deeply and will be hard to wake.

Babies over 3–4 months old enter their deep NREM sleep phase at the start of the night so they should find it easier to connect their sleep cycles and experience a consolidated period of sleep before midnight.

5.

REM SLEEP (RAPID EYE MOVEMENT SLEEP)

REM sleep is vital to the development of the brain and it is the state in which we dream. The body rests and the baby processes what she has seen and heard during the day. Young babies spend a lot of time in REM sleep due to its developmental importance.

As your baby gets older she will start to experience more REM sleep in the second half of the night, which is why babies are likely to be more wakeful in the early hours past midnight – this is when they are in their lighter sleep phase. This can be seen on the diagram on page 25.

TOP TIP

6.

UNDERSTAND HOW MELATONIN CAN INFLUENCE SLEEP

Also known as the sleep hormone, melatonin regulates sleep by telling your body it's night-time and it's time to go to bed. When your baby goes to sleep at night, it's beneficial for melatonin levels to be high as this will help your baby to self-settle. Melatonin is produced primarily in darkness so keep the lights low in the evenings.

7.

UNDERSTAND HOW CORTISOL CAN IMPACT SLEEP

This is the hormone created when the body is overtired and sleep-deprived. It's also known as the stress hormone. If your baby's cortisol levels are high, she will find it difficult to go to sleep. Young babies are very sensitive to rises in cortisol and can become overtired and upset very quickly so encourage good daytime naps to reduce these levels. Too much cortisol can also cause regular night-time waking and early rising.

TOP TIP

8.

SLEEP CYCLES
EXPLAINED

As outlined earlier, sleep is not a static state: we go through sleep cycles throughout the night, experiencing different stages of sleep. A newborn baby's sleep cycles are short. However, by the age of around 3–4 months, your baby's sleep cycles will begin to lengthen and she will start to establish the sleep cycle pattern that will be maintained for life. During daytime naps these sleep cycles tend to be around 40–45 minutes, but at night these will start to extend to approximately 60–90 minutes.

So bearing this in mind, **the fact that babies wake regularly is completely normal – it's nature's way of keeping us safe** – but in order to sleep for extended periods a baby needs the ability to get themselves back to sleep between cycles.

9.

UNDERSTANDING YOUR BABY'S SLEEP CYCLES

On the following page is a diagram which illustrates how a typical 6-month-plus baby goes through a roller coaster of sleep cycles throughout the night, transitioning through various stages of sleep, from drowsiness to light sleep, through to deep (NREM) sleep and experiencing periods of dream (REM) sleep along the way. These are also known as sleep stages 1–3. The brief wakings between sleep cycles can become a problem if a baby or child cannot settle themselves back to sleep alone and require the help of a parent or a feed to get themselves back to sleep again.

10.

DIAGRAM TO ILLUSTRATE THE SLEEP CYCLES OF A TYPICAL 6-MONTH-PLUS BABY

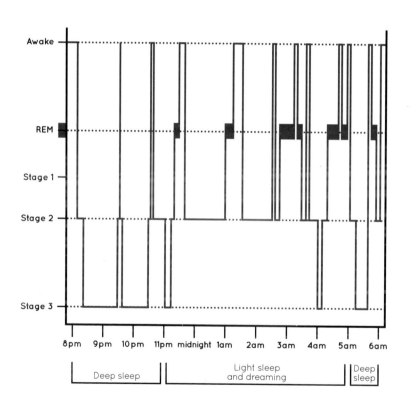

CHAPTER 2

PRE BIRTH AND THE
EARLY WEEKS

INTRODUCTION

If you're reading this book pre birth I'm going to start by focusing on a few things to prepare you for the impending arrival of your little one and offer some tips for when you first come home.

After the initial shock of being told I was expecting triplets, my first thought was: "However will I cope with three babies?!" I had about 7 months to mentally prepare myself for lack of sleep, hard work and exhaustion, so when our babies arrived and we got into a good routine, my reality was actually easier than I had expected. Not always – some days I just had to take it hour by hour – but my forward planning really helped me to enjoy my babies.

Whether you're having a single or multiple pregnancy, preparation is key.

11.

GET ORGANIZED

Get organized just in case your little one decides to make an early appearance. Spend time with your older children, get your hospital bag packed, organize help and fill your freezer with home-cooked ready meals.

Buy plenty of cotton sleepsuits and short-sleeved vests. These are really comfortable for your baby to sleep in and you'll be amazed how many you get through. Avoid buying sleepsuits that go over the head and button up at the back as these can be difficult to get on a newborn baby.

Also purchase a good supply of muslin cloths. Having one over your shoulder when winding baby not only protects your clothes but also protects your baby from your clothing, which may be fluffy or cause baby to itch.

12.

HAVE REALISTIC EXPECTATIONS

As well as getting prepared practically, it's really useful to prepare yourself mentally for parenthood.

The reality is that from birth, life will change and you may have periods of disturbed sleep for some years to come. Even if your baby sleeps through the night from 12 weeks old she is likely to have regressions which may be caused by developmental leaps, teething, illness, nightmares, separation anxiety or issues at school.

Also, one parent's definition of sleeping "through the night" might be that their baby does a 5-hour stretch and another's definition may be a 10–12-hour stretch, so don't compare your baby to others. I will give you all the tools to help your baby to sleep well, gently guiding them into learning how to self-settle. However, there are no hard and fast rules here – every baby is different and, at the end of the day, they will sleep through the night when the time is right for them.

13.

WHAT TO EXPECT POST BIRTH

Think about restricting your guests for a few days or even a couple of weeks and enjoy this special time without the stress of entertaining visitors.

You cannot overestimate how exhausting giving birth can be. Couple the physical effects with hormonal changes and the huge impact this new life will have on your life, and expect to be tired. This is your time for nesting, cuddling up with your new baby and partner and bonding with each other.

If you do have visitors, don't be embarrassed to ask them to wash their hands when entering the house. Try to avoid too many people handling baby, particularly if it's winter as people are more likely to be harbouring germs, and don't be afraid to ask them to help out – they could pop the kettle on or bring a meal to share.

14.

BABY'S FIRST NIGHT AT HOME

Babies are often very sleepy for the first night and you're likely to be in hospital with help and support nearby. By the second or third night, babies sometimes start to realize that they are no longer in the warmth of the womb being lulled by the sounds of mum's heartbeat and those gently soothing, swooshing sounds, and they may suddenly find their voice. This can be worrying if you're a first-time parent but your baby just needs cuddles and reassurance.

If you are breastfeeding she may wish to feed constantly for comfort. This is a normal pattern of behaviour and will help to stimulate your milk supply but be careful to get a good latch every time to avoid damaging the nipples. See Chapter 3. If you're bottle-feeding you may need to give small regular feeds.

15.

OFFER SKIN-TO-SKIN CONTACT

Offering skin-to-skin contact helps a baby to adjust to life outside the womb. It's calming and soothing, and can give your baby the comfort and reassurance she's craving. Baby is stripped down to a nappy and placed on either parent's bare chest, where she will hear the comforting sounds of your heartbeat as well as experience the warmth and comfort of your skin. It provides multiple benefits, including: regulating baby's heart rate, breathing and temperature; encouraging their natural urge to feed, whether breast- or bottle-fed; promoting bonding between parents and their new baby; and, for a mother, encouraging the release of hormones relating to breast-milk supply and breastfeeding.

16.

DITCH THE
SCRATCH MITTS!

Your baby will enjoy touching your skin and having the ability to put her hands to her mouth as she did in the womb to soothe herself. Scratch mitts are therefore better avoided as they inhibit this important tactile and developmental experience. Your baby's nails will be soft when they're newborn but if they have sharp edges you can remove them with a baby nail file.

17.

WHERE SHOULD MY BABY SLEEP?

Current NHS advice is that your baby should sleep in the same room as you for the first 6 months. This is because studies have shown that when babies sleep in the same room but not in the same bed as a parent, the risk of sudden infant death syndrome (SIDS) is significantly reduced. A Moses basket, crib or carrycot is ideal as it can be moved easily from the living area for daytime sleep to the bedroom for night-time sleep.

Babies should always be placed on their back to sleep with their feet at the foot of their cot, crib or Moses basket to prevent them wriggling down under the covers.

18.

BABIES ARE NOISY SLEEPERS!

I'm often surprised at how noisy some babies are when they're sleeping or trying to get to sleep. Some new parents tend to pick baby up and rock them as they think something is wrong but this can be quite normal and the squeaking, squirming and straining may be part of their digestive process, helping to release trapped wind from both ends. Picking baby up can actually wake her. However, if she starts to actually cry and sound distressed, pick her up and put her on your shoulder for a minute as this is often a sign of wind.

19.

DON'T FORGET TO WIND YOUR BABY

Whether your baby is breastfed or bottle-fed it's important to hold her upright after a feed as babies often swallow air when feeding, which can result in discomfort and an unsettled baby. Either sit her up on your lap, supporting her chin and straightening her back, or hold her against your shoulder. You can gently pat. However, usually just a straight back will suffice.

Some babies suffer from trapped wind more than others. If she struggles to burp, try laying her on a flat surface like the sofa or changing mat for a minute then pick her up and put her on your shoulder for a minute and repeat as necessary. The action of laying down and then picking up is a sure-fire way to release any trapped wind.

Another method is to gently cycle baby's legs while they're lying flat. Don't do this too soon after a feed or you may cause her to vomit, but it can be very effective if your baby isn't settling and is showing signs of discomfort.

TOP TIP

20.

KEEP DISTURBANCE TO A MINIMUM AT NIGHT

It's important to keep disturbance to a minimum at night. Keep lights as low as possible when feeding at night. Be prepared with everything you'll need so that you don't have to leave the bedroom with baby. For example, if you're breastfeeding, have your comfortable seating prearranged; if you're bottle-feeding, have a good-quality flask of boiling water and powdered formula on hand in the bedroom or use commercially ready-made milk which can be served at room temperature. Equally, make sure nappy-changing equipment, spare sheets and clothes are readily available so you don't have to spend time rummaging around with the lights on.

By following this advice, your baby should be sleepy and easier to settle after her feed.

CHAPTER 3

ESTABLISHING FEEDING

INTRODUCTION

You may be asking yourself why I'm devoting a complete section to feeding when this is a book about sleep. However, a baby will not sleep well unless they are feeding well, so this is one of the fundamental elements to good sleep. We will look at the importance of establishing a good feeding rhythm whether you choose to breastfeed or bottle-feed.

If you are intending to breastfeed, I would encourage you to attend classes and read specialist books.

21.

BREAST, BOTTLE OR BOTH?

Breast or bottle is personal choice and sometimes there is no choice. Not all mums are able to breastfeed. If you do decide to breastfeed, it's not always straightforward so seek help, support and advice. Be warned, however: advice can sometimes be conflicting. The first few weeks can be challenging but if you can get through the early stages it should get easier and easier.

Some mums choose to combination feed: both breastfeeding and formula feeding. If a baby is born prematurely or has medical issues, expressing breast milk and feeding from a bottle is also an option.

22.

LEARN ABOUT RESPONSIVE FEEDING

Responsive feeding is a two-way relationship between mother and baby. Not only does the mother respond to the baby's feeding cues, but also the mother can offer the baby a feed if she feels she wishes to, even if the baby is not looking for a feed, for example perhaps mum needs to go out or wants to have a sleep, or she may feel the need for comfort herself.

A baby's feeding cues include: crying, rooting (turning head and opening mouth), licking lips, sticking tongue out, sucking on hands, fussing and restlessness.

Your newborn baby will need to feed 2–4 hourly. However, she should be woken every 3–4 hours in the first few days if she hasn't woken naturally. Time your feeds from the start of one feed to the start of the next.

If you are breastfeeding, regular feeding gives the message to your body to produce more milk and it's natural for your baby to sometimes want lots of short feeds in the early days of feeding and particularly in the late afternoon or early evening. This is commonly known as cluster feeding.

If a baby is very sleepy, there is a risk that they will not instinctively wake to feed and will weaken. If you're worried, seek advice.

23.

ESTABLISHING BOTTLE-FEEDING

A newborn baby's stomach is tiny – about the size of a walnut – so bottle-fed babies should initially be fed little and often. Respond to your baby's hunger cues but in the early days do not let her go for more than 4 hours from the start of one feed to the start of the next. Once she is taking a bottle well, you can let her go longer at night but continue with 3- to 4-hourly feeds in the day or feed on demand.

Your baby's appetite will vary at each feed. However, the following can be useful for working out how much formula to make at each feed. Most full-term babies need between 150 ml and 200 ml of formula per kilogram of their body weight every 24 hours (or between 2 fl. oz and 3 fl. oz per pound of body weight). So, if your baby weighs 4 kg she'll probably need between 600 ml and 800 ml of formula over a 24-hour period to satisfy her hunger (for an 8 lb baby, 16 to 24 fl. oz). However, she may want less than this in the first week, as she will only have a tiny tummy.

Respond to your baby's cues and needs and just use the above as a guide.

24.

SEEK SUPPORT WHEN ESTABLISHING BREASTFEEDING

If you are breastfeeding, the first couple of weeks are crucial in establishing your supply. Initially your baby will feed little and often but when your milk comes in (which is usually between days 2 and 5 post birth) the time between feeds will increase.

Ensure that baby has a deep comfortable latch so the breast is properly stimulated to encourage milk production and that she is positioned correctly so the nipple is not being dragged to one side or the other. If you need to unlatch your baby, it's important to break the suction before pulling her off the breast to avoid damaging the nipple. Place your clean finger at the corner of her mouth and gently insert it into her mouth between the gums; once your baby opens her mouth, remove the breast.

If you're struggling with any aspect of breastfeeding, seek support **immediately**. There should be a breastfeeding adviser available in hospital and once you're home you can get help via your midwife, health visitor service, a local support group or a private lactation consultant.

25.

WHAT TO EXPECT WHEN YOUR MILK "COMES IN"

In the first few days your breasts will be producing colostrum, a form of milk that is thick, sticky and often yellowish in appearance. Even though it seems that only tiny quantities are produced, it is rich in calories and antibodies so feeding your baby little and often will deliver these vital nutrients and give your body the message to produce milk.

For most mothers the milk will increase in quantity and begin to change to mature milk between days 2 and 5 post birth. This is generally known as the milk "coming in". One of the signs of this is that the breasts become fuller and firmer.

If baby is feeding well and frequently, this stage should pass without any problems. However, for some this can result in engorgement, with the breasts becoming very full, firm, warm and possibly tender. This can make it difficult for baby to latch.

You can help to manage this by applying warm, wet flannels on to your breast just before a feed, hand expressing to soften the areola before you attempt to latch and massaging any lumps that appear. Try to ensure that your baby fully empties one breast at each feed and then top up with the other if necessary, ensuring that you start with alternate breasts at each feed.

26.

HOW TO ENSURE A GOOD LATCH

"Latch" refers to how your baby is attached to the breast when feeding and is also known as "a good attachment". A good latch promotes high milk flow and minimizes discomfort, while a poor latch can result in low milk transfer and can lead to damaged nipples.

If your baby is spending a lot of time at the breast it doesn't necessarily mean they are getting a lot of milk. Watch and listen for swallowing to check that your baby has a good attachment or latch. Swallowing should be frequent at the start of the feed and less often toward the end. You should see the lower jaw moving up and down rhythmically, hear swallowing and observe your baby take short rests. Toward the end of the feed you may see fluttery, quivery sucking movements which are generally not active feeding.

This is why it's impossible to say exactly how long a baby needs to feed for. A baby who has a good latch and is feeding effectively may take a full feed in 20 minutes but a baby who has a poor latch may feed for an hour or more and still not be full.

27.

WORK ON "ACTIVE" BREASTFEEDING

In these early days of feeding it's important to work on "active" feeding.

Try this:

Breastfeed for about 10 minutes normally. (Babies tend to get sleepier as they feed – it's hard work!) Continue to encourage active feeding for about another 10 minutes but if baby is sleepy use techniques such as stroking her cheek, tickling toes, putting gentle pressure on the breast to encourage milk flow, or opening up baby's clothing as the cool air may help to rouse her.

Wind and change nappy.

Repeat the process either with the first 10 minutes on the same breast if it feels like there's still milk and then the final 10 minutes on the other side, or the full 20 minutes on the second side.

Wind baby well.

With a full 40 minutes of active feeding, your baby should have a full tummy and be ready for sleep, so swaddle her and lay her in her crib and you should hopefully get a good rest before your baby needs feeding again.

28.

MAKE EVERY FEED COUNT!

Whether you are breast- or bottle-feeding, this is so important. If you aim for your baby to get a nice full tummy at each and every feed, she should be satisfied and ready for a good long nap. If baby falls asleep mid feed, change her nappy to wake her up and feed some more! Wind her well during and after a feed and try to avoid getting into a rhythm of snacking.

For breastfeeding mothers this will also help to prevent baby spending all day on the breast, feeding half-heartedly, thus making your nipples sore and you exhausted.

29.

GIVE AN OCCASIONAL BOTTLE TO AVOID BOTTLE REJECTION

Even if you decide to fully breastfeed, giving a bottle of expressed breast milk regularly once your baby is a few weeks old will help to avoid her refusing to drink from a bottle further down the line and will also give mum the opportunity to have a break or a rest if necessary. Wait until breastfeeding is fully established and be aware that if you're replacing a complete feed with a bottle feed you will need to express within a couple of hours of your usual breastfeed time to avoid affecting your milk supply or risking engorgement.

It's not uncommon for an older baby to reject a bottle feed if they are unaccustomed to it. This can be a real problem if mum is unwell, needs a break, or is held up in any way when another person is caring for the baby. Offering a bottle of expressed milk (or formula if you prefer) every couple of days has the added benefit of giving your partner a chance to get involved with feeding.

30.

AVOID A SNACK AND NAP RHYTHM

If your baby is snacking and napping, you are likely to be exhausted and baby will be unsettled. Your baby will not sleep well if they are hungry. The exception to this is if they are failing to thrive (losing weight), in which case they may sleep more so you should be alerted by excessive lethargy.

One of the most common situations, particularly for new parents, is that baby may have a small feed and then fall asleep in their parent's arms. Mum or dad are delighted baby is sleeping and gently lower her into the crib, then 15 minutes later baby is awake and crying!

CHAPTER 4

HELP YOUR NEWBORN BABY TO FEEL SAFE AND SECURE

INTRODUCTION

Meeting your baby's physical and emotional needs, providing a safe, secure and consistent environment along with love, touch and plenty of cuddles will help your baby to feel a strong emotional attachment to their parents or carers.

These are essential requirements for good sleep and a content, happy baby.

It is common for babies to go through unsettled and fussy periods, often in the late afternoon or early evening. This can be due to over-stimulation, wind or digestive issues. Try the techniques in this chapter to help settle your baby.

31.

RECREATE THE WOMB

The best way to calm and soothe a newborn baby to sleep is to recreate the noises, movement and snug environment of the womb.

Babies *in utero* are rocked and swayed and hear the whooshing and gurgling sounds from their mother's body while being cradled by the walls of the womb. You can recreate this environment by using the techniques explained on the following pages – start with the first and add the subsequent ones as necessary depending on how unsettled or distressed your baby is.

32.

SWADDLE YOUR BABY

Swaddling helps to recreate the snug feeling of being in the womb, making baby feel safe and secure, which can help to trigger sleep. It can also prevent your baby waking herself up with the Moro reflex, also known as the "startle reflex". This is an involuntary response present in babies for the first 3 to 6 months.

There is a large variety of styles to consider and there are plenty of online videos to help you with swaddling techniques. Ensure that you do not wrap baby too tightly around the legs and hips as this can cause problems with the hips: your baby's legs need to be able to move into a natural "frog-like" position.

Follow safe practice guidelines, do not use a thick blanket as your baby may overheat and ensure her face is not covered. It's advisable to stop swaddling by 12 weeks as your baby will become more physically active, may begin to roll and may also want to suck on her thumb or fingers to help her to self-settle.

33.

HOLD IN A SIDE OR STOMACH POSITION

Newborn babies tend to feel secure and content on their side or tummy so these are good positions for soothing. Hold your fussing baby in your arms on her side (her tummy to your tummy), or on your chest in a tummy-down position or place her against your shoulder.

If necessary, use the further soothing techniques as detailed on the following pages. Once you've soothed her to sleep, place her down on her back in the safe sleep position as this reduces the risk of SIDS.

34.

SHUSH YOUR BABY TO SLEEP

Shushing loudly or gently depending on how loud your baby is crying can help distract them from crying and induce sleep. Newborns are not used to silence as mum's blood flow makes a loud shushing, whooshing sound *in utero*. Singing songs and lullabies is also calming for babies.

As your baby gets older and more aware of her environment, white noise can be helpful to block out the sounds of you coming to bed, or traffic and general sounds if you live in a noisy location. White noise can be played via a digital device and can vary from womb, heartbeat and shushing sounds to more mechanical sounds like fans and hairdryers. Leave the noise on for the whole sleep otherwise you will find that baby may wake as soon as it's switched off.

35.

ROCK OR GENTLY SWAY

In utero your baby was rocked and jiggled, so it makes sense that babies are comforted by motion. You can recreate this by gently moving your swaddled baby back and forth while holding them in a side position. Ensure the head is supported and just use gentle movements.

Carrying baby in a sling or baby carrier held against your chest can also be a very effective way of comforting her if she is particularly unsettled or upset.

36.

COMFORT SUCKING

Some babies love to suck and find great comfort in it, particularly if they suffer from colic. This is also known as non-nutritive sucking. You can either give a pacifier/ dummy or offer a clean finger to the roof of the mouth. However, it's important not to use a dummy in the first weeks before feeding is established as you may disguise a baby's feeding cues when they are genuinely hungry.

It's very easy to overuse a pacifier so try to keep it for those occasions where you really need it to avoid it becoming a sleep association, where your baby becomes dependent on it to go to sleep. Sleep associations are discussed on page 103.

37.

HAVE PREDICTABLE RHYTHMS

Having predictable experiences throughout your baby's day will help her to feel safe and secure – we will discuss routine later. Even from newborn you can create a regular rhythm to the day. Instead of clock-watching, try to think of it as a sequence of events with a consistent pattern. For example: nap, feed, cuddles and interaction, nap and so on, ending the day with a calming bath before bedtime.

38.

BUILD TRUST

If a baby or young child feels your responsiveness when they need reassurance this will help them to have the security to explore their world knowing that you will respond to their needs. This is why using cry-it-out methods of sleep training from a young age is not recommended. Helping your baby to get to sleep in your presence using touch and reassurance will help build their trust, subsequently improving their long-term sleep patterns.

39.

KEEP CALM

Babies are sensitive to anxiety or stress. An anxious carer can add to a baby's stress, making her harder to soothe. If you are feeling stressed, try to find ways to calm down before interacting with your baby. There are many relaxation methods you can try, but a very simple and effective one is to simply stop, take a deep breath and slowly release it. Repeat this action several times and notice how calm it makes you feel. Alternatively, you could try a change of scenery: take your baby out for a stroll where the exercise and fresh air can work wonders for you. Stress levels can be heightened when you are tired so try to seek help from your partner, a friend or a relative to give you a chance to rest and recuperate.

TOP TIP

40.

HELP YOUR BABY TO FEEL SAFE AND SECURE IN THEIR CRIB

You can't over-cuddle a newborn baby; however, for her to feel safe and secure in her crib or Moses basket you need to put her in it from the start. This certainly doesn't mean never cuddling a sleeping baby in your arms, but if you do that all day, every day and then put her down alone in the crib at night she may not be too happy. Move the crib to the living area during the day or put her down swaddled in the flat cot of her pram and gently rock her back and forth so she starts to feel comfortable sleeping alone but knowing that you are nearby.

CHAPTER 5

TEACH THE DIFFERENCE BETWEEN NIGHT AND DAY

INTRODUCTION

A newborn baby does not know the difference between night and day – she is simply governed by hunger. In fact, newborns are often on an opposite rhythm to you because while in the womb they are rocked and soothed to sleep all day with your movement and voice, and at night, while you are lying still, they wake. It can take a little time to reverse that pattern.

However, you can help your baby to learn to distinguish night from day. The following tips can be used from birth and continued in the long term.

41.

DAYTIME

LIGHTEN UP THE MORNING

For newborn babies, once you are ready to start your day, allow daylight into the room to help differentiate night and day.

For older babies, decide what time is acceptable to start the day – I would suggest that 7.00–7.30 a.m. is ideal but any time after 6.00 a.m. is acceptable, of course, depending on your baby's age and the time they went to bed. Throw open the curtains and use your happy "morning" voice. Allowing daylight into the room will help to suppress your baby's melatonin levels and regulate their body clock. Using your "morning" voice gives a powerful message that day is different to night-time.

42.

DAYTIME
INTERACT AND PLAY

During the day, interact and play with your baby frequently; smiles, laughter, talking, singing, music and touch are essential for your baby's development. She will enjoy the sound of your voice and may even mimic your facial expressions. As she gets older, you can plan more stimulating social daytime activities; for example, baby groups, music and movement sessions, and swimming all help you not only interact in a new way with your baby but also meet and share experiences with other parents.

43.

DAYTIME

GET PLENTY OF FRESH AIR AND DAYLIGHT

Try to ensure your baby is exposed to fresh air and daylight every day by going out for walks or just being out in the garden or the park.

Higher daylight levels encourage the early development of the biological clock, which regulates a number of bodily functions, including the secretion of melatonin, the sleep hormone, an important factor in influencing well-balanced sleep patterns.

44.

DAYTIME

DON'T MINIMIZE DAYTIME NOISE

There is no need to minimize daytime noise around the house. Carry on as normal so your baby gets used to everyday sounds like the radio, vacuum cleaner, washing machine, telephone and voices. You will be surprised what she is able to sleep through.

45.

DAYTIME

ENCOURAGE MORE DAYTIME CALORIES

During the first month, don't let your baby go for longer than 3–4 hours without a feed. Time your feeds from the start of one feed to the start of the next. Gently guide her into taking more calories during the daytime then she will need fewer during the night. After 6 weeks of age, encourage a little awake time between feeds without allowing her to get overtired.

46.

🌙

NIGHT-TIME

HAVE A PREDICTABLE BEDTIME ROUTINE

If you carry out the same sequence of events at a similar time each night, you create sleep cues which your baby will learn to connect with bedtime. This will help her to differentiate between night-time sleep and naptime so she is more likely to sleep for longer periods between feeds.

A key part of the bedtime routine is a lovely calming bath time. Keep the lights low as bright lights suppress the production of melatonin, the sleep hormone. Change her into comfortable nightwear or use a baby sleeping bag or swaddle.

This important part of the day is discussed in detail in Chapter 6.

47.

🌙

NIGHT-TIME

USE BLACKOUT BLINDS

As discussed earlier, daylight suppresses melatonin, so if your baby is exposed to daylight in the bedroom she will find it more difficult to get to sleep and is more likely to wake early in the morning.

For older babies and toddlers you may want to consider buying portable blackout blinds for travelling so you can create a snoozy sleeping environment in any home you stay in.

48.

☾

NIGHT-TIME

ENSURE YOUR BABY'S ROOM IS A COMFORTABLE TEMPERATURE

It is important to ensure your baby's room is a comfortable temperature – not too hot and not too cold – and also check for draughts. An ideal room temperature is around 16°C (61°F) to 20°C (68°F), which allows for baby to sleep with light bedding or a lightweight, well-fitting sleeping bag.

The safest place for a young baby to sleep is in a room with you so you should be able to judge a comfortable temperature. If you're unsure, room thermometers are reasonably priced. If you use blankets ensure they are firmly tucked under the sides of the mattress so they cannot come loose and smother baby's face and do not put a hat on a baby indoors.

In the summer months it can be difficult to regulate the temperature; use lighter bedding and sleepwear, open a window if it's safe to do so and if you use a fan, ensure it's not directed at the baby.

49.

🌙

NIGHT-TIME

BUY A DIMMABLE LIGHT FOR NIGHT FEEDS

In order to keep the light as low as possible for night feeds, thus helping to avoid your baby fully waking, buy a dimmable light. There are many portable rechargeable ones available which are perfect for night-time. Ideally, use a light with a red or orange bulb as white and blue light can inhibit the secretion of the sleep inducing hormone, melatonin.

Keep disturbance to a minimum. Taking baby out of a darkened bedroom into the lounge or kitchen to feed will inevitably involve bright lighting and doesn't help baby to learn to distinguish night from day. If you're worried that night feeds will disturb your partner, who may have work the following day, you can consider your partner sleeping in a separate room if space will allow.

50.

🌙

NIGHT-TIME

BE BORING AT NIGHT

When you're caring for your baby at night, keep interaction to a minimum. Use your quiet "night-time" voice to comfort your baby but do not play or chat.

This tip is equally important for older babies and toddlers. Night-time is not a time for engaging in conversation. Be calm and give quiet but firm instructions at night, such as: "It's sleep time now. See you in the morning."

CHAPTER 6

ESTABLISHING A BEDTIME ROUTINE

INTRODUCTION

A regular and predictable bath and bedtime routine relaxes your baby and helps melatonin levels rise, which in turn will help your baby settle more easily. A routine also creates cues to help your baby to understand the difference between night-time and daytime sleep. Babies learn by association, so they quickly get used to a repetitive pattern and start to expect what comes next.

It's never too early to establish an evening routine. I like to give an evening bath as early as one week old as most babies find it calming and even from this age they seem to sleep better following a bath.

However, if you haven't done this by the time your baby is 2–3 months old, then now is the time to implement it using the following tips.

51.

CREATE A PRE-BATH-TIME TOY BOX

In the build-up to bath time, make space for calm, quiet time. This is particularly important for babies over 4 months old, toddlers and older children. If you're engaging in physical, boisterous play just before bed, your baby's adrenaline and cortisol levels will be high, which is not conducive to sleep.

Create a box of "calm" toys. This should include hand–eye coordination toys like shape sorters, puzzles, simple games and drawing. Bring this box out after teatime so it has some novelty value and engages your baby or toddler. This will help create a calm atmosphere before bedtime.

TOP TIP

52.

AVOID TV AND SCREEN TIME IN THE EVENINGS

Avoid exposing your baby or toddler to television or screens in the early evening as the blue lights from such devices inhibit the production of melatonin, the sleep hormone, basically telling the body that it's daytime, not night-time.

53.

OFFER A "SLEEPY" SNACK

Sleep-friendly foods can calm the mind and boost the hormones that promote good sleep.

Tryptophan is an essential amino acid that helps us to sleep and is naturally present in foods such as dairy products, turkey, bananas and oats, among others. However, these should ideally be eaten alongside healthy complex carbohydrate foods as these cause the release of insulin, which helps tryptophan reach the brain and cause sleepiness.

It takes about an hour for the tryptophan in foods to reach the brain, so for weaned babies and older children, offer a sleepy snack just before heading up to bath. This can be as simple as a glass of warm milk and a banana, a bowl of porridge, a piece of wholemeal toast and peanut butter, or some healthy crackers and cheese. Bananas also contain magnesium and potassium which are natural muscle-relaxants, making them a great, quick and easy sleep food.

54.

KEEP YOUR TIMINGS CONSISTENT

For newborn babies bath time can be flexible but from 2–3 months your bedtime routine should commence around the same time every night and should take no longer than 30–45 minutes. If you make your routine longer than this, your baby will lose focus and you will not benefit from the melatonin increase. By keeping to regular timings your baby will be ready for sleep; if you change it nightly she may be overtired or under-tired at bedtime and may find it difficult to settle. There will inevitably be occasions when the routine gets disrupted but, where possible, try to stick with a regular routine as the sleep benefits are worth it.

55.

ESTABLISH A FAMILY-FRIENDLY ROUTINE

Plan your routine around a time that fits in with your family life and other children. For example, there is no point in bathing your baby, having her all warm, cosy and drowsy, and then your partner comes home from work and wants to play. Your baby is likely to end up overtired and overstimulated.

Bath time is a great opportunity for both parents to be involved. If your partner is not involved in the daytime care then bath time can be their special time. Along with sharing responsibilities, this provides a perfect time for bonding.

56.

TIME FOR BED?

Around 7.00 p.m. for bedtime seems to fit in with many families so that would mean commencing your routine around 6.15–6.30 p.m. but ensuring quiet time before then.

If you prefer a later bedtime and a later start to the day, you might like to aim for 8.00 p.m. and start your routine at 7.15–7.30 p.m.

There is no right or wrong here. In hot countries the day often starts later, a siesta is enjoyed in the afternoon and children stay up late as this is the coolest time of day. Plan your day to suit your environment and lifestyle – just try to keep it consistent.

57.

MAKE BATH TIME A CALMING AND RELAXING EXPERIENCE

Bath time should be calming and relaxing. However, this can be easier said than done.

When there are the needs of other children to consider, try to think of ways to include older siblings and encourage them to be your helpers. If you have multiples or children of different ages, this is a time to accept offers of help; if you're already tired this can be a challenging time of day and, as we have previously discussed, babies may pick up on your stress.

If time allows, giving a post-bath massage can soothe your baby, help her to sleep and has many other benefits, including aiding digestion, improving circulation, reducing crying, and helping you and your partner to bond with your baby.

58.

AVOID RETURNING TO THE LIVING AREA AFTER BATH TIME

Once your baby is a couple of months old, after bath time it's beneficial to go straight to the bedroom. If you go back to the living area, your baby will be restimulated and you will not be taking advantage of the higher melatonin levels. This is key to your baby having the best opportunity to self-settle.

Organize yourself before you start bath time so you have everything you need to hand, including nightwear, milk and a book for story time.

TOP TIP

59.

GIVE A SPLIT FEED BEFORE BED

My preference is to offer a split feed around bath time: half a feed in the living area before heading to bath and then a small top-up feed after the bath. Alternatively, from around 4 months you may wish to give the complete feed pre bath to separate feeding and sleeping and avoid your baby developing a feed-to-sleep association.

The advantage of a split feed is that your baby will have an enjoyable bath without being too hungry and she is likely to take a bigger feed overall. The post-bath top-up feed should be just a smaller, calming feed. Try to avoid your baby falling asleep while feeding, and then read a short story or sing a lullaby, and after a cuddle put your baby to bed, drowsy but awake.

60.

SLEEP CUE WORDS

When you put your baby down for a sleep, whether during the day, night or in the middle of the night, say the same words each time. Something like: "Night night, <name>. It's sleep time now. I love you and I'll see you in the morning/in a little while." Then give a kiss and a cuddle.

Sleep cue words are powerful and reassuring. Babies and children learn by association. You are gently saying what you expect of them, affirming your love and telling them that you're coming back. Your partner, the grandparents, nanny, childminder or whoever is caring for your baby should use the same comforting words.

CHAPTER 7

NAPS

INTRODUCTION

Daytime naps are so important. It's a myth that if babies sleep during the day they won't sleep at night – the opposite is true! Naps are a good teaching time and sleep encourages sleep. If your baby is well rested she will find it easier to go to sleep at night, be more content and have a healthier appetite. If you restrict naps, your baby will be overtired and her cortisol levels will increase.

The timing of naps will affect your whole 24-hour cycle. If you're trying to put your baby down to sleep when she's overtired or under-tired it will be a battle. It's a fine balance which needs fine-tuning for a good night's sleep. To add complications, a baby's nap needs change as they develop.

61.

CONSISTENCY IS KEY

Up to the age of around 3 months old, your baby's day can be a flexible sequence of events. However, once the circadian rhythm, better known as the body clock, starts to mature, babies and children will respond well to routine to keep their biological rhythms in harmony.

If you put your baby down for her naps at a similar time each day, you will find that she is ready for sleep and should start to settle quickly. If you were to change your bedtime each day, you would find it difficult to fall asleep; the same is true for your baby, so when it comes to napping, consistency is key.

62.

LOOK FOR SLEEP CUES

These can include:

- Staring
- Loss of interest in people and toys
- Decreased activity
- Being less vocal
- Burying her face into your chest
- Rubbing eyes
- Pulling ears
- Yawning and stretching
- Whining and crying.

Sleep cues are sometimes very subtle – don't wait until your baby is overtired to put her down for a nap.

63.

KEEP A NAP DIARY

The secret to good napping is getting the spacing between each nap right. This is where a sleep diary is beneficial. This can be a smartphone app, a printed sleep and feed diary or a simple notebook. Writing down your baby's nap times and lengths will help you to look for patterns and learn to understand your baby's rhythms.

64.

PREPARE FOR NAPS

Newborn babies will sleep in the living area near you during the day. However, once they are 3–6 months old, you may find that they are more disturbed by the noises around them, especially if you have other children.

For older babies, create a mini-nap routine with sleep cues. For example, after some gentle, quiet play or lullabies, go to your baby's nursery or a quiet area, read a short story, maybe say night night to the cuddly toys, close the curtains together and settle her into her cot, gently explaining that it's sleep time and say your reassuring sleep words. Parents quite often have difficulty in getting their babies to nap in their cots during the day and end up taking them for a walk or a drive at every naptime. This is acceptable in the short term for creating a regular sleep pattern but try to encourage a sleep in the cot, crib or Moses basket at least once a day, ideally at lunchtime. If your baby is not keen, be persistent and keep trying.

65.

DAYTIME SLEEP CYCLES

From 3–4 months old, babies' daytime sleep cycles tend to be around 40–45 minutes in length so naps can be 1 or 2 sleep cycles, i.e. 45–90 minutes, sometimes longer at lunchtime. Anything less than 40 minutes does not provide your baby with the full physiological benefits that deeper sleep offers, so if your baby is having lots of catnaps or short naps she is not experiencing fully restorative sleep.

66.

THE MORNING NAP

If you put your baby down for her first nap too early in the day, you may encourage early rising. The same problem can happen if you allow this nap to be too long. The reason for this is because an early, long morning nap will compensate for a 5.00 a.m. wake-up, thus reinforcing it.

From 3–4 months old, the ideal length of the morning nap would be around 45 minutes, and if you're aiming for a 7.00 a.m. start to the day your baby should be ready for her morning nap by about 9.00 a.m.

67.

THE LUNCHTIME NAP

Aim for this nap to be a minimum of 2 sleep cycles, which is approximately 90 minutes. Because this nap is in the middle of the day it will not affect the morning wake-up time or the time your baby goes to bed. This nap should be nicely restorative and can be up to 2.5 hours maximum.

Once your baby is 6 months old and weaned on to solids, ideally this nap will be taken after lunch, around 12.00 p.m. or 12.30 p.m., and ideally it will be in the cot in a darkened room.

68.

HOW TO EXTEND THE LUNCHTIME NAP

It's quite common for a baby to only sleep for a 45-minute cycle at lunchtime but it's worth persevering toward a minimum 90-minute nap.

Try the following:

- Work on getting your baby to self-settle at the start of the nap.

- Ensure she is not napping for more than 45 minutes in the morning.

- If she consistently wakes after 40–45 minutes, ensure that you pause for 5–10 minutes to give her the opportunity to get herself back to sleep.

- If the pause doesn't work, try shushing, patting and soothing her.

- If all else fails, pop her in the pushchair or sling and try to get her back to sleep on the go; even though this is a sleep association, your aim is to reinforce the pattern and for her to get used to sleeping for at least 1.5 hours and then hopefully she will start to do this naturally without your intervention.

If none of the above works don't be despondent; you can do everything in your power to encourage sleep but you can't force it. Tomorrow is another day.

69.

THE LATE-AFTERNOON NAP

If you put your baby down for her afternoon nap too late in the day, you may have problems at bedtime, as your baby will be under-tired. Around 4.00–4.30 p.m. is an ideal time for approximately 30–45 minutes, aiming for her to be awake by 5.00 p.m. for a 7.00 p.m. bedtime. As she gets older, a short catnap of 10–20 minutes is often all that is required in the late afternoon depending on how long she slept at lunchtime.

This nap can sometimes be quite tricky so it's an ideal time to go out for a walk with her in the pushchair or a sling or baby carrier. Also, as it's close to bedtime, having a cot nap can trigger night/day confusion so is best avoided.

Babies usually drop this nap at around 6–8 months old.

70.

NAP SCHEDULES

———

I don't like to offer prescriptive routines as every baby and family are different. However, if you're aiming for a 7.00 a.m. to 7.00 p.m. day, I would generally aim toward the following nap schedule from around 4 months old. It can be adapted to suit your lifestyle.

- 9.00 a.m. – 45 minutes
- 12.00–12.30 p.m. – 1.5–2.5 hours
- 4.00–4.30 p.m. – 30–45 minutes (as your baby gets older this may reduce to just a 20-minute power nap)

You can adjust these timings around your baby and her needs, but work toward a rhythm of a short morning nap, a long lunchtime nap and a short afternoon nap.

The first nap that your baby will drop will be the late-afternoon nap and this generally happens between 6–8 months depending on how long she sleeps at lunchtime.

The next nap transition is usually between 14 and 18 months, when her naps will reduce from 2 naps to 1 long nap straight after lunch.

By the time your toddler is 3 years old, she may no longer need a daytime nap if she's sleeping solidly at night, but some toddlers will continue to have a 45-minute nap until they're around 4 years old.

CHAPTER 8

THE 3–4-MONTH WINDOW OF OPPORTUNITY

INTRODUCTION

Given the fact that sleep cycles extend and melatonin levels increase from around 3 months of age, your baby should be able to sleep for more extended periods at night by this time. In addition, at this age, the circadian rhythm, better known as the body clock, is maturing. This is the 24-hour sequence of biological cycles which influence patterns of sleeping, waking, rest, hunger, activity, body temperature and hormones. Babies and children respond well to routine as a means of keeping these rhythms in harmony. This is the ideal time to guide your baby into a healthy routine, to establish regular feed times and nap times, to follow a predictable bath and bedtime routine and encourage self-settling.

TOP TIP

71.

AVOID THE 4-MONTH SLEEP REGRESSION

This is a commonly discussed sleep regression, but it is actually a developmental progression! At around 3–4 months of age, your baby's sleep pattern begins to mature and they start to sleep in sleep cycles. Your baby will be rousing approximately every 60–90 minutes during the night in between her many sleep cycles. Sometimes this may present as just a slight stirring and other times it will be a full wake-up. This can result in a sleep regression for babies *who haven't learned to self-settle* and are dependent on some sort of prop or sleep association to get to sleep. This is possibly the most important fact about your baby's sleep that you need to grasp: it is normal for babies to wake regularly during the night – this is nature's way of keeping us safe – but the key to prevent them from fully waking is for them to have the ability to settle themselves back to sleep again without the need for a parent to create the same conditions that got them to sleep at the start of the night. For this reason it is important to start to encourage self-settling and establish a regular but flexible routine round 3–4 months of age or earlier.

72.

PUT YOUR BABY TO BED DROWSY BUT AWAKE

Drowsy but awake means putting your baby down when they are calm and relaxed and aware of going to sleep in their crib or cot. This is the key to your baby sleeping well and there is no right or wrong time to start. If your baby is well fed and comfortable she may be happy to go into her cot drowsy but awake from newborn. Be guided by your baby. It's never too late to start. If you are reading this book when your baby is a few months old use the techniques in Chapter 9 to help you achieve this.

73.

KEEP CONDITIONS CONSISTENT

———

Alongside the ability to self-settle, your baby needs to find herself in exactly the same conditions when she partially wakes as when she fell asleep at the start of the night. Having the security that all is well and that her conditions haven't changed will give her the confidence to drift off again and only fully wake if she is hungry or has other needs.

After 3–4 months old, if, for instance, she falls asleep being rocked in your arms and then she wakes between sleep cycles alone in her bed no longer being rocked, she may fully wake, distressed by the changed environment, and need to be rocked back to sleep again. This is like you going to sleep in your bed and waking up on the floor!

Similarly, if your baby falls asleep in her cot with the musical mobile playing, there will be noise, movement and possibly a light show, but when she rouses during the night it will be silent, still and dark. Instead of feeling safe and secure, she may be disturbed by her change in conditions and cry for attention.

74.

UNDERSTAND SLEEP ASSOCIATIONS

Helping your baby to discover her own way of self-settling is a fundamental step in encouraging her to sleep through the night. If your baby has fallen asleep dependent on any kind of prop, she may wake repeatedly during the night and need to be helped back to sleep again.

Common sleep associations or props:

- Feeding to sleep – breast or bottle
- Rocking
- Cuddling
- Patting
- Music
- Motion – car or pushchair
- A dummy/pacifier

75.

AVOID A FEED-TO-SLEEP PATTERN

Once your baby is over 6 weeks old and is spending more time awake during the day, try to create a rhythm whereby she is not having a feed just before a nap. This is key to avoiding her developing a feed-to-sleep association. Feed your baby shortly after she has woken from her nap rather than just before she goes back down for her next nap. This has the added advantage that it should encourage her to take a good, full feed as she won't be falling asleep while feeding.

A positive sleep–awake pattern to follow is:

- Nap
- Feed
- Play/interaction/cuddles
- Nap

If you need to offer a top-up feed before the long lunch nap, try to ensure that you don't feed-to-sleep. Look at a picture book or sing a lullaby to break the association between feeding and sleeping.

76.

LEARN ABOUT THE PROS AND CONS OF USING A DUMMY AS A SLEEP AID

The pros and cons of using a dummy as a pacifier are a matter of constant debate. If you choose to use one it's best not to introduce it until feeding is established otherwise it may disguise hunger if your baby is not feeding well. If you have a particularly unsettled baby and decide to introduce a dummy once feeding is established, try to only use it when essential rather than to just keep your baby quiet and try not to use it as a permanent sleep aid.

To avoid it becoming a dependence, it's best to try to wean baby off it by 3 months old and encourage her to learn to settle without the need to suck on a dummy. If you decide to keep the dummy, there is often a stage of sleep regression where baby is dependent on it to fall asleep and stay asleep and may need to have it put back in several times throughout the night.

Once your older baby becomes more dexterous, encourage her to put her own dummy in her mouth, so she doesn't depend on you to do it for her, or you can purchase a specially designed small, safe, soft toy which has Velcro hands and feet to attach dummies on to and is easier for baby to find in the cot.

77.

DON'T BECOME A HUMAN DUMMY

In the early weeks of breastfeeding it is highly likely that your baby will fall asleep on the breast as breastfeeding can be very tiring and breast milk contains sleep hormones. It can be a comfort to both mum and baby to use breastfeeding as a sleep aid at this time. However, as she gets older, if she is *dependent on nursing as a sleep aid* there is every possibility that she will need to nurse regularly throughout the night in order to connect her sleep cycles. It's much easier to break this habit earlier rather than later.

Once your baby is 6–8 weeks plus, try the following:

During daytime feeds, when your baby has finished breastfeeding, gently unlatch her from the breast, wind her and then have some quiet play, interaction time and cuddles before she is due her next nap.

When you're giving the last feed before bedtime, try not to allow her to fall asleep on the breast – it's unavoidable when she's tiny but as she gets older, wind her and indulge in a gentle activity, such as looking at a book together, before settling her into the cot. In creating a break between breast and sleep, you will disassociate feeding and sleeping, the most common sleep association.

78.

DON'T MEET EVERY EMOTIONAL NEED WITH FOOD

Demand feeding, also known as responsive feeding, means feeding your baby whenever she signals that she's hungry – usually by crying, rooting or sucking on her hands – rather than according to a set schedule.

However, babies cry for all manner of other reasons – they're wet, they're tired, they're in pain, they're bored, they're uncomfortable – so it's important to establish why your baby is crying and what she needs rather than quell every cry with food.

79.

LET YOUR BABY HAVE A VOICE

Crying is your baby's only form of communication. If you immediately quell every cry, how can you understand what your baby is trying to tell you?

- Is she hungry?
- Is she bored?
- Is she uncomfortable?
- Does she have wind?
- Does she need a nappy change?
- Is she too hot or too cold?
- Is she unwell?
- Is she trying to connect sleep cycles? (This may often involve a little crying or grizzling.)

Try to differentiate between her cries. Babies have different cries for different needs. Is she actually crying because she's distressed and hungry or is she letting off some steam and trying to settle herself to sleep? For clarification, I'm not suggesting you leave your baby to wail – just that you respect her voice.

TOP TIP

80.
PAUSE!

Babies can be noisy when learning how to connect sleep cycles, with sounds varying from crying, moaning or grumbling. It is very easy for a parent to react too quickly to their baby's stirs because they don't want their partner to be disturbed or they may be worried that a sibling will be woken. However, these quick reactions can actually wake the baby when, if she were left for a few minutes, she may resettle herself. Instead, pause, observe and listen. Rushing to every stir or grizzle means you're basically connecting her sleep cycles for her, never allowing her the opportunity to learn to self-settle, which will subsequently encourage regular waking. If her grizzle becomes a cry of need, then, of course, you attend to her.

The feedback I get from parents is that allowing a pause is one of the most powerful and simple things that really makes a difference to their baby's long-term sleep habits.

CHAPTER 9

TEACHING YOUR BABY TO SELF-SETTLE

INTRODUCTION

When you put your baby to bed, whether it's for naps or night-time sleep, they need to feel safe, secure, loved and nurtured. Newborn babies may need lots of help to settle to sleep. As your baby gets older, teaching them to self-settle will give them some sleep independence and will mean that they are more likely to resettle themselves at night in between sleep cycles. The earlier you start to encourage your baby to self-settle, the easier it is – however, it's never too late.

In this chapter we will look at appropriate settling techniques depending on age.

81.

GO THROUGH THIS CHECKLIST FIRST

Before embarking on any sleep-teaching techniques, remember to take a holistic approach and check the following first:

- Does your baby have a sleep association? If so, what is it?
- Is your baby having regular naps, and are the lengths and times age appropriate?
- Do you have a regular, predictable bath and bedtime routine?
- Is your baby eating well during the day?
- Is your baby in good health?

It's important to ensure that there are no wider issues that need to be addressed before helping your baby to learn to self-settle.

82.

0–2 MONTHS: ANYTHING GOES!

This is a time for bonding and getting to know your baby. She may need a lot of comfort and cuddles in these early weeks along with help to settle to sleep and to connect her sleep cycles. However, do give her the opportunity to sleep in her crib or Moses basket during the day and then she will be happier in there at night. Although it's lovely to hold a sleeping baby, she needs to feel comfortable in her own space, so giving early opportunities for this will be beneficial in the long term.

83.

2–4 MONTHS: GIVE GENTLE REASSURANCE

Some babies go through stages where they like to sleep upright on a parent's chest and this can become an established habit but with some perseverance it can be reversed. When she's ready for sleep, has a clean nappy and is not hungry, cuddle her until she is drowsy and then settle her into her crib, put a firm, comforting hand on her for a minute or two, then step back and see if she settles. She may cry a little; if this crying escalates, try to soothe her with one of the gentle trust-building techniques on the following pages, which reinforce the message that she is loved and safe.

84.

2–4 MONTHS: PAT YOUR BABY TO SLEEP

Gentle, rhythmic patting can mimic the sound and rhythm of a mother's heartbeat in the womb, which is calming and relaxing for babies. This is a great technique for settling your baby in their cot or crib.

Place your baby in her crib, ideally in a darkened room, gently roll her on to her side, supporting her tummy with one hand. With the other hand, rhythmically and firmly pat her bottom in an upward motion. It may help to sing a lullaby, shush or play white noise too. Once baby is asleep, roll her on to her back for safe sleeping.

When your baby gets more proficient at settling in this way, start to reduce the patting over a period of days and then maybe just put a firm, reassuring hand on her.

85.

2–4 MONTHS: PICK UP, PUT DOWN

If your baby's cries are escalating and she cannot be calmed by shushing and patting, pick her up and comfort her until she is calm and drowsy but not asleep. Put her back in her cot, and repeat this cycle as necessary until she is asleep. This method requires time and patience, and for some babies the picking up and putting down may be overstimulating.

This technique can also be very effective when teaching a baby to sleep flat when they have become used to only napping in a baby carrier or sling. Put baby in the pram and walk around the garden or house for a minute, even if she is crying. If she is still crying, pick her up and hold her against your shoulder, walk around the garden or house for another minute and then return to the pram for a further minute. Repeat as necessary until baby falls asleep in the pram. This method is a real winner for reluctant nappers!

86.

4–6 MONTHS PLUS: TECHNIQUES FOR SETTLING OLDER BABIES

If you have not taught your baby to self-settle before now, this is your window of opportunity to do so. I would suggest you start with the night-time sleep following your bath routine to take advantage of your baby's higher melatonin levels. It's important to be consistent. Your baby can only respond to the sleep cues you give her so if you change tack every couple of days she will just become confused.

As before, try to settle her in her cot, saying your reassuring sleep words. If you're unable to get her to sleep using the techniques outlined on the previous pages then follow the gradual retreat method on the next page. The crucial thing is to see it through until sleep is achieved. If your baby protests, just stay with her, continue to settle and comfort her – almost cuddle her in her cot if you need to.

Try to resist picking her up. However, if she is distraught and you need to, once she is calm and before she is asleep, lay her back down and start again. You aren't abandoning her to her cries and she will not feel unloved as you're staying with her until she is fully asleep. Do the same at every sleep situation and each time she achieves sleep in this way it should be easier the next time.

87.

GRADUAL RETREAT: STEP 1

Gradual retreat is my preferred technique for helping young babies, toddlers and older children to settle to sleep. If your baby has become dependent on props to get to sleep, try this kind and gentle process.

Many babies get into the habit of falling asleep while breast- or bottle-feeding, so the first degree of separation from this will be to rock her to sleep without feeding. Once she has mastered this, the next step is to help your baby to go to sleep in her cot using whatever intervention works to help soothe her. It can be anything from just a firm, reassuring hand on her, to patting, shushing and singing lullabies. Anything goes as long as they fall asleep in their cot with you by their side.

Once your baby is comfortable to go to sleep with your help and soothing, you need to move to the next degree of separation otherwise she may form a dependence on your presence to get to sleep.

88.

GRADUAL RETREAT: STEP 2

Your next step will be to use less intervention: maybe just offer an occasional pat and shush, or take away either the touch or the voice element. The retreat continues every couple of days until you are ready to just sit next to her cot and then over time you move your chair further and further away.

If you're teaching this from a young age, you will move through the steps more quickly. Be mindful that your goal is to teach your baby to settle without your presence. You're aiming to lay her in the cot after a cuddle, say your reassuring sleep words and leave the room.

89.

ENCOURAGE YOUR PARTNER TO BE INVOLVED

When it comes to teaching your baby to self-settle, it cannot be a "one size fits all" approach. All babies are different so you need to find the soothing "key" for your baby. Some will be calmed by your presence and some may be overstimulated by your presence so you need to choose an approach that works for you.

Both parents should share in this settling process so your baby isn't dependent on only mum settling her. In fact, if you're a breast-feeding mum you may find that your partner is more successful as your baby will associate you with nursing.

90.

BE CONSISTENT, PERSEVERE AND BE POSITIVE

If you've been trying multiple methods to get your baby to sleep but with no success, it could be the very fact that you've used too many methods that's causing your baby confusion. Make a plan and stick with it.

Even though sleep teaching can be time consuming, persevere and see it through. It's not always plain sailing as some babies can be quite determined but if you do it for half an hour and then give up, you're just teaching your baby to resist sleep for half an hour before you rock her or feed her to sleep. If you're consistent you may be amazed how quickly you see results.

Be positive! If you dread putting your baby down for her sleep she will sense your anxiety. Put her down confidently and expect her to sleep. Once you have a routine in place and she learns to self-settle she should love going to sleep.

CHAPTER 10

ROUTINE, NIGHT FEEDS AND FEEDING YOUR OLDER BABY

INTRODUCTION

As I've already said, feeding and sleeping go hand in hand. A baby won't sleep well if they are hungry. Feeding can also impact sleep in a negative way, particularly if your baby starts to take the majority of their calories at night instead of during the day, so in this chapter we will look at establishing a routine, feeding your older baby and weaning off night feeds.

91.

ESTABLISH A ROUTINE

Babies love routine! In the early weeks you may have been feeding responsively and following your baby's cues, but once your baby is around 8–10 weeks old, try to establish a regular daytime feed and nap rhythm to avoid your baby becoming overtired. Instead of clock-watching, learn your baby's rhythms by keeping a sleep and feed diary. Think of it as a sequence of events with a consistent pattern that is repeated throughout the day and establish a routine tailored to your lifestyle and situation. If it seems daunting at first, focus on setting the morning wake-up time and first nap of the day and be consistent with bedtime; once these are established you will find it easier to work on the middle of the day. Some degree of flexibility as opposed to a rigid routine works well.

At 12–16 weeks, you can start to aim toward a routine with more structure, with naps and feeds at the same time each day. This will avoid your baby becoming overtired or over-hungry and she should generally be more content. It also means that you as a parent can structure your day around your baby's patterns.

92.

DON'T DREAM FEED YOUR BABY

Some parenting advisers recommend "dream feeding" (feeding your baby while she is still asleep) at around 10.00 p.m. or 11.00 p.m., before the parents go to bed, with the aim of getting a longer stretch of uninterrupted sleep. I disagree with this method. By dream feeding you're in danger of creating a habitual hunger at that time and you're interrupting her natural rhythms, disturbing her sleep-pattern development and feeding her when she isn't hungry. Moreover, at this time of night she is in the deep NREM sleep phase, a time of important physical development, so it's not the best time to be stimulating the digestive system. If you allow your baby's natural rhythms to develop, the length of time she sleeps should gradually increase, especially during this period of deep sleep where she should find it easier to connect her sleep cycles.

93.

HAVE AN EARLY NIGHT

In my mind, a much better solution than dream feeding is for the parents to have an early night so that they can achieve a decent period of deep sleep before being woken. There's an old saying: "One hour before midnight is worth two after." The origin of this is that we experience our deep, restorative, NREM sleep at the start of the night, so take advantage of achieving this at a time when your baby is also in her deep sleep phase and you're less likely to be disturbed.

Remember: this difficult period of adjusting to your baby's sleep patterns is such a short time in the grand scheme of things that a little compromise on your part as a parent can really pay dividends in the long term.

94.

THERE'S NO NEED TO WAKE YOUR BABY AFTER A NIGHT FEED

When your baby wakes for a night-time feed, keep interaction to a minimum, give the feed (either breast or bottle), wind and settle her back into the cot as quickly as possible. If she is asleep there is no need to wake her before putting her back into her cot.

Once she's a couple of months old, only change the nappy during the night if necessary. However, in the early weeks, changing the nappy mid feed can help to wake her up enough to take a proper feed rather than a half-hearted one which will not result in a long period of sleep.

95.

TO FEED OR NOT TO FEED?

As your baby gets older, don't always assume she needs a night feed each time she wakes. If she fed 2 hours previously, she shouldn't need feeding again. Try to resettle her using the methods discussed in Chapter 9. It may be difficult at first, but with consistency it will get easier. Feeding her back to sleep is a short-term, quick-fix solution, which may ultimately reinforce the night-time waking.

If your baby is settling independently at the start of the night she should sleep for longer and longer stretches during the night, naturally dropping night feeds and only fully waking between sleep cycles if she is genuinely hungry.

96.

WEANING OFF NIGHT FEEDS

Between 4 and 6 months old (depending on what country's guidelines you are following), you will start to wean your baby on to solids. Once weaning is successfully established, she should no longer need milk during the night, providing she is in good health. If you've taught her to self-settle from a young age she may well have stopped waking for night feeds long ago. If she is still waking this is probably out of habit.

Regular night feeding can create a negative cycle where your baby is filling up on calories during the night and not needing to eat so much in the day. Once you wean off night feeds, you should see her appetite improve during the day. If you have a particularly hungry baby or your baby has medical issues, or if you have any doubts, consult your GP, paediatrician or health visitor before reducing night feeds.

97.

HOW TO WEAN A BOTTLE-FED BABY OFF NIGHT FEEDS

For a bottle-fed baby you can increase the time between feeds or gradually reduce the volume of milk given over a period of nights. For example, you can reduce the volume by 15–30 ml (0.5–1 fl. oz) each night until you are down to a feed of 30–60 ml (1–2 fl. oz) and then stop altogether. If necessary, use gradual retreat or another settling technique, as detailed in Chapter 9, to soothe your baby back to sleep.

98.

HOW TO WEAN A BREASTFED BABY OFF NIGHT FEEDS

There are two methods to reduce night feeding. The first is to decrease the amount of milk you are giving your baby at each feed. For a breastfed baby, gradually reduce the number of minutes offered at the breast over a period of nights and once you're down to a couple of minutes, stop altogether. If necessary, use gradual retreat or another settling technique, as detailed in Chapter 9, to soothe your baby back to sleep.

The second method is to increase the interval between feeds. For example, if your baby is feeding every 3 hours, increase the time between feeds to 4 hours for 2 nights and then 5 hours for 2 nights and so on. Once again, use a settling technique to help soothe your baby back to sleep if necessary.

99.

CREATE A POSITIVE SLEEP ASSOCIATION

Encourage your baby to form an attachment to some sort of comforter. This could be a safe, small, soft toy, which will inevitably end up having a name such as "a lovey". You are aiming for this comforter to become a sleep trigger, so each time you place it with your baby she may caress it, rub it between her fingers and become soporific. This is what your baby will turn to for comfort in the middle of the night when she wakes briefly between sleep cycles and it will help her to self-soothe.

Current SIDS guidelines advise that you should not place soft toys in the cot in the first 12 months but you can familiarize your baby with it before then by giving it to her to hold when you're having a cuddle or she's in her pram or car seat. Once she is old enough to have her comforter at sleep times, place it in her hand as you lay her in the cot and, if you're lucky, it will become a positive sleep association which is portable, always giving your baby a feeling of comfort and security, particularly when you're in unfamiliar surroundings.

100.

DON'T COMPARE YOUR BABY TO OTHER BABIES

There is no magical age at which all babies sleep through the night. It depends on so many factors: her health, her size, how well she feeds and if she has learned to fall asleep independently. Some babies sleep through the night much earlier than others. If your baby is still having a night feed at 6 months this may not be a problem for you but if she's waking every 2 hours then you need to work out why and address the issue.

Above all, make the most of this special time, enjoy your baby and be mindful that this period of disturbed sleep is relatively short.

TROUBLESHOOTING TIPS

Sometimes it may be just a snippet of advice that makes all the difference to your baby or toddler's sleep so in this bonus chapter I want to reiterate a few points.

The first step when reviewing sleep issues is to analyze why they're happening. Sometimes the answer is obvious and parents know where things are going wrong but are too tired to address it and consequently do anything to get a bit more sleep, thus reinforcing the problem. Making the effort to put things right will produce long-term benefits for the whole family.

Once you commence you need to be consistent. You can't have "one-off" nights where you bring your baby into your bed because it's the easy option and is quite nice! That's unfair on your baby.

1.

WORK OUT WHY

Before you can address any issue with sleep, you need to analyze why it's happening. Often it's a combination of things. Work out what they are, make a plan, write it down and give yourself small, realistic goals. Remember that two teachers are better than one so ensure that you, your partner and anyone else caring for your baby are doing exactly the same as you.

Some reasons for sleep problems are:

- Hunger
- A sleep association (see Tip 74)
- The timing and lengths of naps – a very common reason for sleep problems (see Chapter 7)
- Inadvertently rewarding the waking
- Day/night confusion
- Too hot or cold
- Being uncomfortable – use soft, cotton nightwear with no buttons at the back and no logos which may be irritating to sensitive skin
- Teething
- Illness
- A milk allergy or intolerance
- Reflux and Silent Reflux
- Obstructive sleep apnoea (enlarged tonsils)
- Nightmares
- Night Terrors

2.

RULE OUT HUNGER

———————

One of the most common reasons for a newborn baby being fussy and unsettled is as simple as this: hunger. Newborn babies' feeding patterns may not fit in with your idea of a schedule. Try to go with the flow for the first few weeks. Trust your baby's feeding cues, even if they have recently fed. Some babies like to cluster feed in the evenings, whether they're breast- or formula-fed. This does have its advantages: they seem to instinctively "tank up", which often results in a good period of sleep at the start of the night. While you're recovering from the journey of birth, take advantage of this by going to bed at the same time as your baby.

3.

DON'T REWARD
THE WAKING

This tip is aimed at babies over 6 months old, toddlers and older children.

A child's inappropriate behaviour is often unintentionally rewarded. A prime example of this is when a baby or toddler is repeatedly waking in the night and the parent's response to this is to bring their little one into bed with them. It's a sure-fire way to ensure the waking never stops! What a fabulous reward for night-time waking: getting to snuggle up in the parental bed.

Sometimes this behaviour starts after a change or break in routine, maybe a holiday or the arrival of a new baby. If you're reading this book as a new parent and if co-sleeping is not your parenting choice, try to avoid ever doing it in the first place and then your child won't know it's even an option.

Other rewards may include offering an older baby or toddler a bottle or a breastfeed in the middle of the night, creating a night-time habitual hunger, or going downstairs at 5.00 a.m. and putting the TV on or playing. All will reinforce the waking.

To break this habit you need to help soothe baby back to sleep in her cot using gradual retreat. For older children this can be combined with a star chart or marbles in a jar for positive behaviour and a reward system.

4.
RIDE OUT THE REGRESSIONS

Sleep regressions can happen for a number of reasons: a developmental progression (physical, psychological or emotional); teething; illness; a holiday or house move; the arrival of a new baby, to name but a few.

If your baby is in a good routine and is not dependent on negative sleep associations or props to get to sleep, you just need to patiently work through the regression and try not to develop negative habits.

If your baby is poorly they will need love and cuddles and if it's necessary to be with them at night it's better to stay in their room than move baby into yours. Don't worry about your routine being disrupted; poorly babies need lots of healing sleep.

5.

EARLY RISERS

Early rising is a common issue; it is frustrating and exhausting for parents and can be difficult to resolve.

Common reasons for early waking are:

Rewarding the waking – rewards can come in various forms: milk, food, cuddles, taking baby into bed with you, playtime, television. All of these will reinforce the early waking thus establishing it so it becomes habitual.

Timing of daytime naps – if your baby is over 3 months old the longest nap of the day should be at lunchtime. If she has a long early morning nap this will compensate for an early wake-up and thus perpetuate it.

Light – Ensure there is no daylight filtering around the edge of the curtains. Light suppresses the sleep hormone, melatonin, and will therefore contribute to early waking.

Early sleep phase – Be realistic with your expectations. If your baby goes to sleep at 6.30 p.m. and wakes at 5.30 a.m. she will have achieved a solid 11 hours of sleep so is unlikely to resettle. Either have an early night yourself to accommodate the early start to the day or gradually try to reset her body clock so she goes to sleep 30 minutes later in the evening.

Late sleep phase – this may seem counterintuitive but if your baby goes to sleep too late at night they are likely to wake even earlier in the morning! Our bodies release cortisol and adrenalin when we are overtired. This can cause your baby to have trouble settling and can cause night-time wake ups and an early start to the day.

6.

BE PREPARED THAT THINGS MAY GET WORSE BEFORE THEY GET BETTER

You may be trying to change well-established habits so be aware that things may get worse before they get better. Change takes time to establish. You should see improvements within a few days if you take a consistent approach but be prepared that to completely turn things around can take weeks depending on the situation. For this reason, choose a good time to begin: when you are well, your baby is well and you don't have any travel or holidays coming up.

Also be prepared for "test" nights or days. You may have turned a corner and seen a great improvement and then have a difficult night. This is a common pattern but if you see it through, maintaining your consistent approach, this is often followed by real improvement.

7.

DON'T CONFUSE NIGHTMARES WITH NIGHT TERRORS

Nightmares occur in REM or dream sleep so they usually happen in the second half of the night. They are most common in young children and reach a peak around 3–6 years when the imagination is developing. They can be distressing for the child so you will need to offer comfort and reassurance as a young child can confuse a dream with reality.

Night terrors occur in deep NREM sleep so they're usually present in the early part of sleep and sometimes within half an hour of going to sleep. Night terrors are very disturbing for the parents as the child may be screaming, crying or moaning, and may be wide-eyed, may get out of bed and be inconsolable. Although this can be deeply distressing for the parents, it is unlikely that the child will have any recollection of the experience so do not wake them as this is likely to cause further upset.

One of the causes of night terrors is being overtired so a constant bedtime and a good routine of daytime naps that are age-appropriate, will help to balance the biological clock.

8.

TWINS, TRIPLETS AND MORE

As a mother of triplets, I would say the key things that worked for me were routine, being ultra-organized and trying to stay one step ahead of the game.

Try to create a consistent pattern of feeding and sleeping, and once your babies have reached a healthy weight, if your health visitor or paediatrician is in agreement, you can allow them to sleep for longer periods at night. If one wakes to feed, I would suggest you feed them all to keep them in a consistent pattern. Establish a set bedtime for your babies, encourage them to self-settle and don't worry too much about them waking each other. Multiples generally don't seem to be too bothered by their siblings' cries. You can choose to sleep your multiples in the same cot (co-bedding) or allow them to sleep in separate cots.

The early weeks will be very tiring so try to sleep when your babies sleep, and even if you only have time for a "power nap" in the day, you will feel better for it. If your babies' cots don't fit in your room, set up a bed in their room and if you have a partner, take turns in doing the night feeds, when possible.

Young babies can often get very fractious in the early evening, needing extra cuddles and soothing. If possible, try to get some help at this time; however, if you are alone, simple bouncy chairs are helpful as you can rock them with your feet while simultaneously soothing another baby. Try to get out at least once a day, as light and fresh air help to develop your babies' biological day/night cycles.

9.

LOOK AFTER YOURSELF!

We have focused on tips for helping your baby to sleep better but in order to implement positive parenting you need to think about self-care too. If you have the luxury of help, try to have a bit of time to yourself every now and then. Pamper or treat yourself.

Keep up with your friends who can be a great support network. If you are feeling low, talk about it. It is natural to have baby blues around day 5 post birth; however, if you feel the baby blues are continuing or coming back it is a good idea to discuss it with your GP or health visitor. There is so much help available for mums with postnatal depression but until you talk about it, it is difficult for people to offer you the help you need.

Take a nap! There is little time to spare as a busy parent but even a short power nap or 10 minutes of mindfulness can be incredibly restorative. Give it a go!

10.
EXPECT SUCCESS!

Be positive and expect success. At the risk of sounding repetitive, I can't stress this enough. The key elements for success are positivity, time, repetition and consistency!

ACKNOWLEDGEMENTS

I would like to thank Dr Ella Rachamim, community paediatrician at Royal Free Hospital Trust, Dr Hugh Selsick, Consultant in Sleep Medicine and Psychiatry at Royal London Hospital for Integrated Medicine, and Beth Graham, midwife and lactation consultant, for their time and expertise checking my book and ensuring I provided medically correct information.

For reading my early drafts I am grateful to Sarah Wheeler, midwife and Norland nanny, and to Annabel Howard, for reading it through the eyes of a new mum. Thank you to my very patient editors, Anna Martin and Claire Plimmer. Also to all the lovely mums, dads and babies I have worked with over the years, who have given me a wealth of hands-on experience.

Finally, of course, to my own family for their love and support; Chris, my husband and my fabulous children Alex, Max and Evie, who I am immensely proud of.